Legal Dis

MW01268669

This book is not in.

disease. If you have a health problem, medical emergency or general health concern, you should contact a physician or qualified health care provider for consultation, diagnosis, and treatment. The information contained in this work has not been evaluated by the FDA (Food and Drug Administration) or any other official government body.

The information contained within this work is based on the experience and research of the author. It is not intended to be a substitute for seeing a qualified health care practitioner and it is to be used for educational purposes only. By continuing with the program you recognize that despite all precautions on the part of the author, there are risks of injury or illness which can occur because of your use of the aforementioned information and you expressly assume such risks and waive, relinquish and release any claim which you may have against the author/vendor, or their affiliates as a result of any future physical injury or

Table of Contents

Welcome To Shin Splints Secrets! 4

What Are Shin Splints? 6

What Causes Shin Splints? 10

Pain Reduction Strategies 20

Corrective Stretches and Exercises 28

Condition Specific Action Steps 37

Tips For Preventing Shin Splints...41

Conclusion..43

Bonus Report: How To Pick the Perfect Shoe........................45

Welcome To Shin Splints Secrets!

First off, I want to thank you for putting the faith in my approach for treating and preventing shin splints.

In this manual I'm not going to waste a lot of your time with "filler" info. You want to know what to do – exactly how to get permanent relief from your shin splints in the shortest period of time – and that's what I'm going to deliver to you (while saving you the tedious chore of reading a textbook).

This is stuff that has taken me YEARS to figure out.

This program is broken down into three parts.

First you'll learn about what shin splints are and what's REALLY causing yours...

Secondly, you'll learn about the most effective pain relief techniques to reduce the swelling and inflammation that you're experiencing fast.

Finally, you'll learn treatment and prevention strategies that will address the ROOT causes of your shin splints and eliminate them once and for all.

I recommend you read this guide in order, and most importantly, don't stop using what you learn until your shin splints are GONE!

Many people make the mistakes of learning something and then saying "I get it" and not taking ACTION on it, don't be one of those people!

These strategies WILL work for you and eliminate your shin splints for good very quickly as long as you stick with them.

When you do you'll see dramatic improvements in your condition, and with a bit of luck, your shin splints will be gone within just a week or two. You may have tried some treatments in this past and you may of suffered with shin splints for years. But you're about to learn methods that work, and things that will just "make sense"... and when you put it to use and see the results you're looking for I have only one request.

Now let's get started...

What Are Shin Splints?

Recent studies indicate that approximately 13.1% of all runners suffer from shin splints, as well as a variety of other athletes and people engaged in all types of sports.

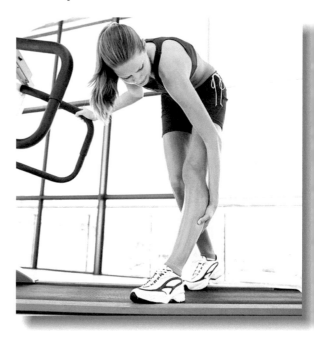

It's pretty simple to get relief from shin splints, but that relief tends to last only until the next time you're running, jumping, sprinting or engaged in your favourite sport or physical activity.

And many athletes end up in a never ending cycle of pain, frustration and temporary relief... but others manage to eliminate them once and for all...

So what's the difference that makes a difference? Why is it that some people manage to get rid of shin splints for good whilst others struggle with them for years?

Well I believe I have the answer to that question... but before I can tell you what it is we need to get very clear on what shin splints are and the understand the basic anatomy involved.

Shin Splints Basics

Shin Splints is a "gutter term". It's used by both athletes and medical professionals to refer to pain along the shinbone (tibia) – which can be caused by a variety of overuse injuries and lower leg problems.

NOTE: there are several more serious conditions that cause pain in this area, namely compartment syndrome and stress fractures. (Which we'll discuss in a later section)

Shin problems are generally due to a number of causes such as tight calves, inactive glutes or poor running form just to name a few. The problems are then made worse by the fact that when you run you increase your body's effective load by 2.5 times.

In other words, if you weigh 180lbs you're actually putting 450lbs of effective weight on your bones and joints when you're running. It's not hard to see that when your body has weaknesses and imbalances already that all that extra stress can cause some injuries quite easily. To better understand Shin Splints let's have a look at the anatomy involved...

Anatomy

Let's get into it, the lower leg is made up of two bones. The larger one is called the tibia and the smaller, thinner bone on the outside of the lower leg is called the fibula.

There are two main muscles involved in shin splints which are pictured to the right.

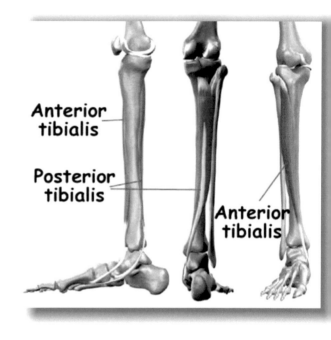

The first is the **tibialis anterior** which is located on the front of the shin, which flexes the ankle bringing the toes to a pointed up position.

The second is the **tibialis posterior** which is located inside and behind the tibia, which stabilizes your foot and flexes the ankle the opposite direction, bringing your toes to a pointed down position.

The Two Types Of Shin Splints

The first and most common type of Shin Splints which is called Posterior Shin Splints aka Medial Tibial Stress Syndrome (MTSS) which is a specific type of shin splints which causes pain in the lower 2/3's of the shinbone, on the inside edge of the shinbone.

The second type of Shin Splints which is associated with the tibialis anterior is Anterior Shin Splints which causes pain on the front of the leg, which is especially intense when lifting your toes off the floor while your heel is still planted on the ground.

What Causes Shin Splints?

In this chapter you're going to learn about the causes of shin splints and how to tell which ones are causing yours.

But before we get into that, let's get clear on what makes the difference between those who get permanent relief from shin splints and those who continue suffering... most people who are trying to treat shin splints use mainstream treatment techniques that fail because they don't target the root causes of shin splints, but instead target the main symptom... which is PAIN.

The pain you feel is not the enemy... it's a desperate message from your body telling you that something is wrong inside.

What's wrong is that your body has one or more of the major underlying causes that you're about to learn about, these are the major factors that contribute to shin splints, and once these problems are addressed, your shin splints will be gone for good.

There are many possible causes of shin splints, and while this section cannot possibly cover all of them it does cover the most important factors so grab a pen and paper, and go through this section carefully to identify what's causing yours.

1) Incorrect or inappropriate training methods or surfaces.

Shin splints are most likely to appear when you increase the intensity, frequency or duration of training. This is especially true if changes are abrupt. Training on hard surfaces like concrete or uneven surfaces like snow or sand can also be a catalyst for shin splints – especially if you've never done this type of training before.

This is where honest self assessment comes in. Have you increased the intensity, frequency or duration of your training recently? Have those increases been abrupt? Have you been training on hard or uneven surfaces? Are you giving your body enough time to recover?

From now on, avoid abrupt increases in training difficulty. It's very important for the health of your body that you increase the amount of training you do and how intense it is gradually, If you start to experience any pain, you slow down or cease the activity causing you pain immediately.

As a general guideline, avoid increasing the intensity or duration of your workout by more than 10% per week to help avoid shin splints and other injuries.

Over the next week or two the corrective exercises that you'll be doing will strengthen the muscles, tendons and ligaments in your lower leg, which will help your body be more fit to handle the strain put on it by training.

2) Muscular imbalances or lack of flexibility

Muscle imbalances, inflexibility, weakness and instability are all factors which can lead to the onset of painful shin splints.

The body is an amazing fine-tuned machine, but it's important to understand that over a lifetime we have taken on postural or other repetitive habits that have tightened up certain muscles and have weakened others.

The three most common ones that lead to shin splints are inflexibility of the calf muscles, over-pronation of the foot and weak or inactive gluteal musculature, unfortunately there are many more and it's virtually impossible to cover them all.

That being said, the three main ones are covered in some depth below and the general flexibility and strengthening exercises later in this book should take care of the majority of other possible problems without you having to worry about them at all.

Problem #1 – Weak or Inflexible Calves

A physiotherapist friend of mine once told me that "if there's any problem that's synonymous with shin splints than its weak or inflexible calves". Both in my own experience and in helping many others recover from this condition I've consistently found this to be true.

The calves consist of two main muscles, the soleus and the gastrocnemius. Both of these muscles connect to the foot and when they become tired, weak or inflexible this can compromise the strength and stability of the ankle, which can and most of the time will contribute to aches and pains in the shins as well as many other forms of injury.

So, it goes without saying that of the corrective exercises later in the book there are several dedicated towards stretching and strengthening the calves.

To check if weak or tight calves is a likely factor in your shin splints, take this quick test.

- Do your calves ever feel tired, tight or sore during exercise?
- Do your calves ever feel tired, tight or sore after exercise?
- Do your calves stay tired, tight or sore for long periods after exercise?

If you answered yes to one or more of these questions, then you'll most likely benefit greatly from the calf exercises later in this book.

Problem #2 - Over-pronation of the foot:

Over-pronation, or flat feet, is a common problem that involves a person's arch collapsing upon weight bearing. This motion places a lot of stress on the tendons and ligaments in the ankle which can trigger inflammation, as well as potentially causing shin splints or other foot problems.

This problem generally occurs in people who have flat feet, or people who have low or collapsed arches. To check the health of you arches, take this quick test.

The Wet Test

This is a simple test you can do at home. Make sure to do this test on both feet as it's not uncommon for the result to vary. Here's how it works, you need to wet the bottom of your feet and step onto a piece of paper or any surface that will show an imprint of your foot. Check the wet footprint after about 15 seconds, and compare it to the diagram below.

The Normal Foot: has a "normal arch" and will leave a wet footprint that has a flare, but shows the forefoot and heel

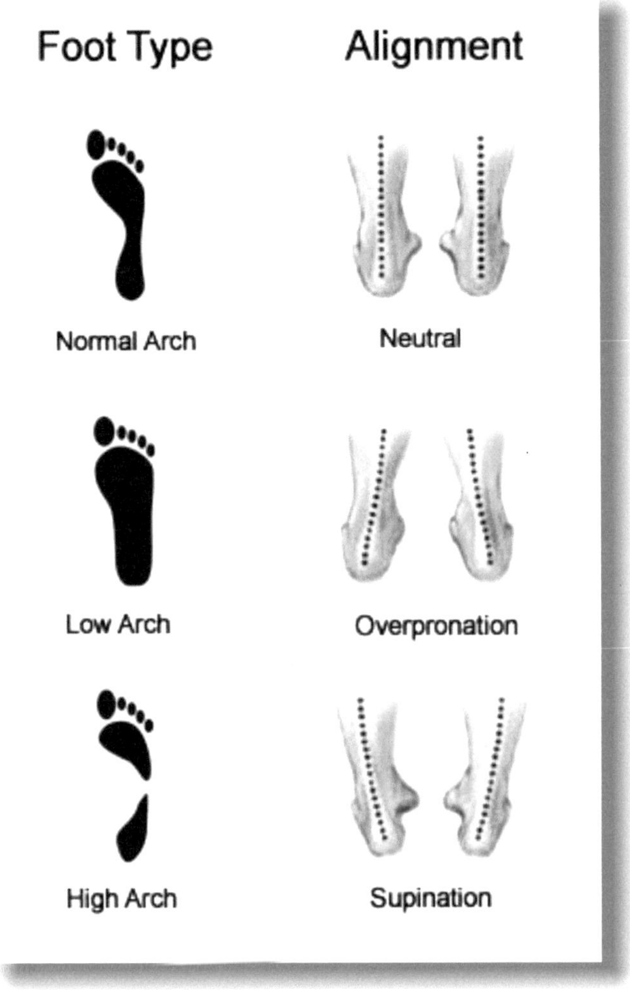

Foot Type

Alignment

Normal Arch

Neutral

Low Arch

Overpronation

High Arch

Supination

connected by a broad band like the top picture to the right. A normal foot lands on the outside of the heel and pronates (rolls inwards) slightly to absorb shock. If you have this type of foot congratulations, you can move on to the next section!

The Flat Foot: has a "low arch" and leave a print which looks like the whole sole of the foot. A flat foot overpronates meaning it usually lands on the outside of the heel and rolls inwards (pronates) excessively which can cause shin splints and many other overuse injuries.

The High-Arched Foot: has a "high arch" and leaves a print showing a very narrow band or no band at all between the forefoot and the heel. A high arched foot generally supinates or underpronates, because it doesn't pronate enough, it's usually an ineffective shock absorber which can also lead to injuries.

Problem #3 – Weak or Inactive Glutes

Your glutes are actually the strongest muscles in your body, that being said most people's glutes are either not firing at all or are very weak.

This is mainly due to sitting down on a chair for 8-10 hours a day which is a lifestyle problem that's common to many of us. Sitting for long periods of time often makes the hip flexors tight and overactive, which deactivates the glutes.

Weak glutes cause the hamstring and quadriceps muscles to overcompensate, making you far more likely to overpronate your feet, which can contribute to shin splints. Inhibited gluteal muscles also lead to tight iliotibial bands, also known as ITB syndrome, and patello-femoral pain, or runner's knee.

The good news? It's relatively easy to reactivate your glutes if you have this problem, so let's try figure out whether you do have this issue.

The first question to ask yourself is simply do I sit in a chair for 6 hours + per day?

If the answer is "yes", then chances are you have this problem to some extent and will benefit from doing the additional exercises for weak or inactive glutes that are included in a later chapter.

3) Poor shoe/equipment selection

It may sound simple and like it isn't a big deal, but getting the right shoe can be about as difficult as finding the right person to be your mate for life. Ok, maybe that's a slight exaggeration but it's seriously important, everyone's feet are different and getting the right fit is critical.

A client of mine had his professional soccer career ended by a pair of bad shoes. You need this piece of equipment to work properly while you run, or you'll find yourself injured and in pain

- Most running shoes don't last longer than 500 miles without breaking down.
- They'll wear down even faster if you weigh over 250lbs.
- To tell if your shoes are worn out, look at the mid-sole. If there are two or more creases over top of

each other, then your shoe has likely lost over 50% of its ability to support your foot.

Action Step: I've written a full bonus report on *"How To Pick The Perfect Shoe"*, be sure to read it after you finish reading this main guide. Don't worry, it's a quick read! =)

4) Poor Running Technique

Poor running technique is the final common cause of shin splints, it increase the impact and consequently the stress on the tendons and ligaments in your lower legs, Here are a few pointers that should get you running with decent form:

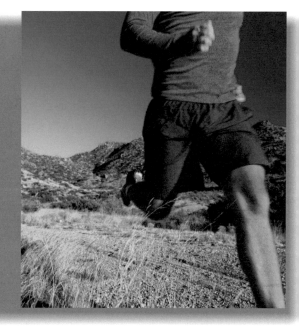

- Do not cross your arms over your body as you run, this is inefficient and a waste of energy. Also be sure not to elevate your shoulders and tighten up; running is all about being loose and having rhythm. Instead try to keep your shoulders relaxed and make sure your arms are pointed forward, but not too stiff.

- Keep your back upright; be proud of yourself when you run. Have a *slight* forward lean but not from the hips.

- You should aim to land softly on the heels and then propel from the toes. However, a common error is to take steps that are too large, this forces you to push from the heels and not the toes when propelling forward. Another common error is to run on the balls of your feet; an effective way to build speed but not easily sustainable.

- Aim to point your toes forward as you run, all too often I find people run with their feet pointed outwards or inwards.

Get those down and you should avoid any unnecessary injury due to poor running technique, you'll also find that once you get the form down, you'll be able to run further and will feel less soreness than usual.

Pain Reduction Strategies

Before we get into treating and preventing your shin splints, it's very important to implement some or all of the pain reduction strategies listed below.

RICE Method

By far the most effective pain relief technique for shin splints is the RICE method. This treatment method is an acronym for rest, ice, compression and elevation. When used recovery times are usually shortened, pain and swelling is minimized. It's important to note that the sooner this method is used, the more effective it is.

How to apply RICE

Rest: Rest is vital to protect the injured area from further strain or injury. A sling or brace is a good choice to keep the limb immobilized.

Ice: Ice is excellent at reducing inflammation and increasing blood flow which helps with nutrient delivery and waste removal which are both key to healing injuries.

There are many methods for applying ice, a plastic bag filled with crushed ice is great, but using cold packs, bags of frozen peas or blocks of ice are all great too.

Direct contact with the skin can cause frost bite or ischemia, so it's important to wrap the ice in a towel before you apply it to the injured area.

A good method for applying ice is using it 10-20 minutes every two hours in the first 24-48 hours. That being said, it depends on the individual and how long they are comfortable with applying the ice for. Just remember that if you feel any pain or discomfort (however slight) it's time to remove the ice.

Compression: Compression helps limit and reduce swelling, which can delay healing. It also provides support to the area to prevent further injury. An easy way to compress the area of the injury is to use a elastic compression bandage bought from any good pharmacy. If the wrap feels too tight or you feel throbbing make sure to loosen it.

Elevation: Keep the injured area elevated above the level of the heart as much as you can. This helps reduce swelling, if you're sitting use a chair and a pillow to help elevate the injured limb and if you're lying down prop your foot up on one or two pillows.

The above information takes care of the first 48 hours. Follow the above advice and you'll cut your recovery time by days, if not weeks.

Two VERY Powerful Pain Relief Techniques

These options take a little more effort and are more inconvenient but as far as pain relief techniques go, they not only provide the most relief, but they are actually amazing at kick-starting your body's natural healing mechanisms.

Note: Use them instead of the "conventional" icing techniques in the previous section.

Pain Relief Technique #1: Ice Dipping

Ice dipping creates a huge circulatory effect that causes your body to bring a rush of nutrients and blood into the area. This gets rid of pain FAST and gets rid of inflammation faster then anything else out there.

Here's how to do it...

1. Fill up your tub half full with water, add a bunch of frozen bottles of water or a big bag of ice to get the water ICE COLD.
2. Adjust the height of the water to your convenience then dip your lower leg into the ice water, submerge it all the way to your knees.
3. Hold it in there for 10 seconds, by then you should be desperate to pull your legs out otherwise the water isn't cold enough...

4. Finally, dry off and walk around for a bit. Wait at least 5 minutes then repeat the process 3-5 times.

I dare you, try this today, you'll see for yourself that this is by far *the most powerful pain relief technique you've ever used!*

Pain Relief Technique #2: Ice Massage

Not quite as powerful as the first technique but still darn good, ice massages force cold deep into your muscles and bones which enhances circulation, flushes out the bodies inflammatory response and if you press a little harder, it also breaks up any scar tissue.

Here's how to do it...

1. Buy some paper cups, fill them with water and put them in your freezer
2. Pull out a cup and tear off the top half inch or so.
3. Massage the exposed ice into the most painful areas of your shins... you'll KNOW you've found the right spot when you're on it... you'll likely feel a sharp pain there.
4. For a minimum of 5 minutes, push the ice into the painful area and up and down your shins. Keep moving around, don't let the ice sit in one spot too long.

Do this at least 3 times a day, if your skin gets numb from the cold it's time to stop.

Stop Exercising

If you are currently exercising, it's very likely that what you are doing is contributing to the problem and possibly making it worse. So the first thing you need to do is to stop exercising for at least three days or until you've seen a decrease in your level of pain and have begun the treatment program.

When you begin to add the exercise or activity back into your routine, you need to start slowly and be aware of how your body is responding to it. If you experience pain slow down or stop, don't let stubbornness or ego get in the way of listening to your body.

Remember, what' most important at this point in time is that you address your imbalances and that sometimes means limiting or even avoiding a sport, exercise or activity you enjoy for a short period of time.

Short Term Use Of Painkillers

While I don't recommend them often, there are times when you might want to use an over-the-counter or prescription pain killer or anti-inflammatory for a short period of time if your pain is unbearable.

If you do use a painkiller like Advil, Nurofen or Ibuprofen then a word of caution is necessary... Use these drugs for no more than a few days, these drugs are called non-steroidal anti-inflammatory drugs (NSAID's) and though they are handed out like candy, prolonged use has very serious side effects like confusion, dependence, lethargy, respiratory illness, stomach bleeding just to name a few...

Your goal should be to use them for 3 days at a time (at most) and get to the point where you don't need them at all as quickly as possible.

Drink More Water!

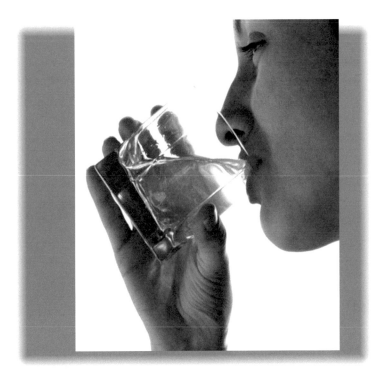

Something like 70% of the U.S. population lives in a chronic state of dehydration.

And NO, Milk, soda, coffee, juice and teas don't count as keeping yourself hydrated!

Even if you think you drink enough water, you probably don't.

Think of yourself as a sponge, the wetter and squishier you are the more resistant you are to injury for many, many reasons. The body needs water to recover from stress, aid with the flexibility of muscles and tendons and to repair tissue and cartilage damage. And that's barely scratching the surface of why water is important to your body, long story short... drink more water.

So how much water is enough?

Most experts recommend eight, 8oz glasses throughout the day... but in my opinion that should be the minimum... *try for more!* The key is to drink water throughout the day and not just at meals or one particular time. I recommend drinking two glasses as soon as you wake up and keeping a large bottle of water with you constantly to sip on.

Massage Therapy

Working with a skilled massage therapist or physio can be a huge help both in recovering from shin splints and ensuring that you never get them again.

Even a bad massage is better than no massage, it gets the blood flowing through the affected area, loosens up the muscles and ultimately helps you feel better faster.

A highly skilled massage therapist if you are fortunate enough to find one can work with you to keep not only your shins healthy but your entire body so it's definitely something I'd recommend.

Corrective Stretches and Exercises

In this section you'll learn a set of general exercises designed to stretch out and strengthen all the muscles and ligaments in your lower leg as well as condition specific action steps used to treat the particular dysfunctions that you identified in the previous sections.

It's recommended that you start performing the exercises and stretches daily in the order we show them... and be sure to be consistent.

Note: Never do the strength exercises before running or exercise.

General Strength & Flexibility Exercises

Exercise #1: Wall Calf Stretch

Stand a little less than arm's distance from the wall. Step your right leg forward and your left leg back, keeping your feet parallel. Bend your right knee and press through your left heel. Hold for 10-15 seconds and switch legs.

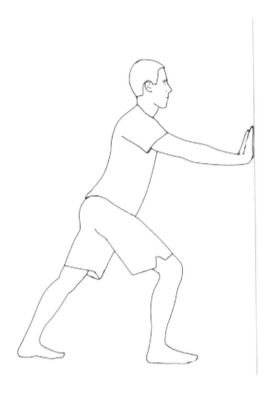

Exercise #2: Kneeling Curb Stretch

Place your toes on the edge of a curb or step, and alternate hanging your heels off toward the floor whilst slightly bending your knees. You'll feel a stretch in the lower section of your calf and the bottom of your foot. Hold for 10-15 seconds.

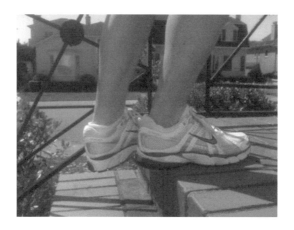

Exercise #3: Seated Shin Stretch

Kneel on both knees with your buttocks over both heels and feet extended back. Slowly sit down on heels – or as far as you can go toward them, it shouldn't hurt. Try not to sit between ankles and avoid this stretch if your suffer from knee problems. Hold for 20-30 seconds and repeat 5 times.

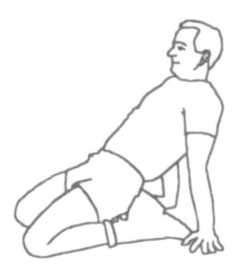

Exercise #4: Standing Shin Stretch

Stand with your toes of the left foot on the floor on the outside of your right foot. Bend the right leg to push your ankle towards the ground. Hold for between 10 and 15 seconds, swap legs and repeat 5 times.

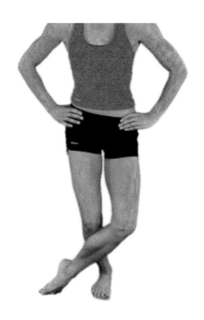

Exercise #5: Weighted Toe Ups

Take a towel and sit on a chair with your feet on a smooth surface. Place the towel on the ground and use your toes to grip the towel and practice lifting it up. Repeat about 100 times. This will help develop the supportive muscles in the bottom of your foot and the front of your shin.

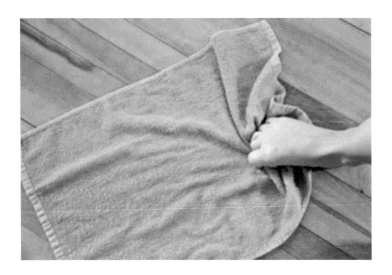

Exercise #7: One-Leg Standing Calf Raise

Place the ball of one of your left foot on the edge of a curb or step and hook your right foot ankle around your left as shown in the picture. Slowly let the heel drop as far as possible. This is the starting position. Slowly raise the heel up as high as possible. Pause, then slowly lower the heel down. Repeat this movement for 20-30 reps for each foot.

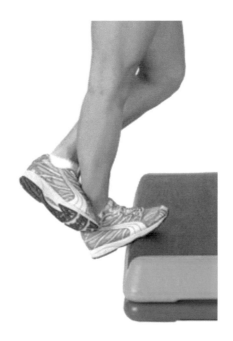

Exercise #7: Toe Walks

Stand on your toes on flat ground and start walking across the room. Walk for 2 sets of 50 steps 25 steps for each leg, for a total of 100 steps. This will help strengthen your calves and ankle as well as actively stretching the shin.

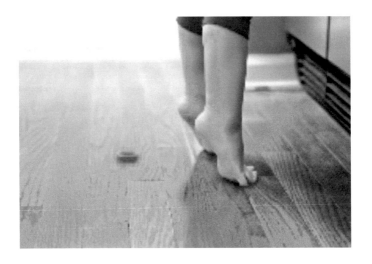

Exercise #8: Heel Walks

Stand on your heels on flat ground and start walking across the room. Walk for 2 sets of 50 steps 25 steps for each leg, for a total of 100 steps. This will help strengthen your shins and ankle as well as actively stretching the calves.

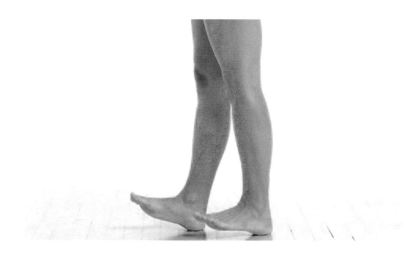

Exercise #9: The Foot Strengthener

Sit on a chair with your feet lifted slightly off the ground and point your toes in the air. Start moving your feet simultaneously to spell the alphabet from A to Z with your toes. Repeat 2 times for each leg. This will help develop the supportive muscles in your foot and ankle. This exercise might sound stupidly simple, but it rocks... if you only do one thing, then do this.

Condition Specific Action Steps

Recommendations For Strengthening Weak or Inactive Glutes

Exercise #1 Toes in Glute Squeeze

Begin standing, turn both feet inward, to get your toes as close together as you can. Slowly, contract your glutes as much as you comfortably can. It is best if you keep your hands on your glutes to feel for the contraction; in the beginning there may be very little if any contraction at all.

Hold for 3-5 sec; repeat 10-15 times, perform at least once per day...

Exercise #2 Bridge Both Single and Double Leg

Begin lying on your back, both knees bent, feet on the floor with arms at your side for support. Slowly push down using your glutes with both feet to life your hips off the floor. Once in the bridge position you can make the exercise more difficult by holding the bridge position and extending one leg and then alternating which leg is extended. The goal is to keep your legs and trunk in a straight line holding at the top position for 3-5 sec. Slowly lower and repeat.

Repeat 10-15 times; perform at least once per day...

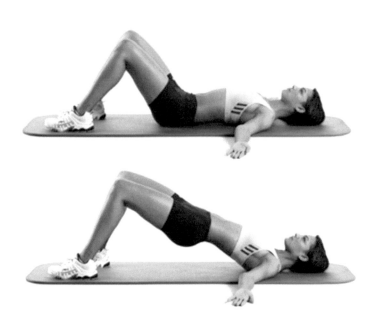

Bridge (both legs).

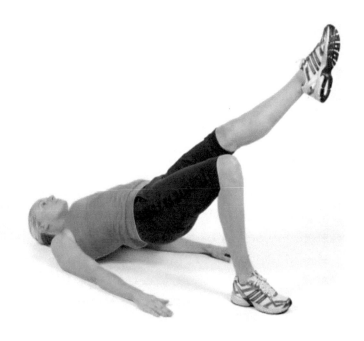

Bridge (single leg).

Recommendations For Correcting Over Pronation of the Foot

Recommendation #1

A good **treatment for over pronation** is professionally fitted and supportive shoes. Shoes should have ample support and cushioning, particularly through the arch of the foot. Without proper shoes there may be additional strain on the tissues in the foot, which greatly contributes to shin splints

Most good running shoe stores will be able to help you choose the right shoe and you can learn much more about this extremely important topic in the bonus report on "How To Pick The Perfect Shoe" included with this program.

Recommendation #2

If you have flat feet then a **well fitted orthotic device** can provide the necessary support to the foot and help restore the proper biomechanical position. Orthotics fit inside of your shoe to provide a platform for your foot to rest in, while in the shoe. You may say "my shoes have arch support!". The truth is, most manufacturers (99%) spend a whole .50 cents on their insoles.

I would **recommend finding a professional podiatrist** in your local area who can create a custom orthotic to suit your foot. The other option is a company called "Super Soles" that has produced a patented cheap shoe insert that runs about $35 and will last over two years. I can only speak from experience in saying these have helped a lot with my shin splints!

Tips For Preventing Shin Splints

Getting rid of shin splints is easy when you know the right things to do. The advice in this chapter will review many of the tips that you've learned so far as well as give you a few new tips and strategies for preventing the reoccurrence of painful shin splints once and for all and helping you build a stronger, faster and healthier body than ever before.

Stop Exercising If You Feel Pain

If at any time you start to feel pain, stop your workout, take a few days and avoid aggravating your shin splints. If you continue to push yourself through the pain you could end up with a more severe injury that sidelines you for even longer.

Cross Training

Just because you've stopped running doesn't mean you can't bike, swim or do yoga in fact I highly recommend you pick a form of exercise that doesn't stress your shins and do it. Not only does this keep you fit, it also aids your recovery by evening out muscle imbalances and strengthening tendons and ligaments that aren't usually used in your regular sport.

Start Slow And Go Easy

To avoid reoccurrence start slow and increase the overall intensity of your training very gradually. Aim to never increase the intensity or duration of your exercise by more than 10% per week.

Warm Up

Always warm up your body directly before any exercise by walking for 3-5 minutes, doing the shin stretches in the exercises sections, and doing some ankle, knee and hip circles.

Workout Surfaces

Walk or run on a soft and even surface to avoid injury upon your return to physical activity.

Walking Barefoot

Hang on a sec, "get great shoes and then walk barefoot?", have I gone crazy? Not quite, when running, exercising or playing sport wear shoes but when you walk around the house or do low impact activities try and walk barefoot as much as possible, and even barefoot on your toes or on your heels as per the exercises in the previous chapters. The feet were designed for barefoot walking so this "natural" way of walking will allow you to strengthen all the tendons and ligaments and avoid further problems.

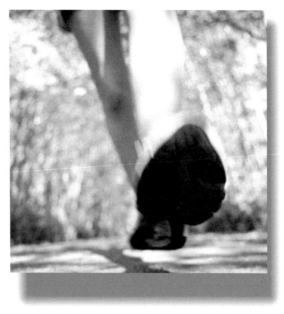

Conclusion

I hope you enjoyed reading this guide as much as I enjoyed writing it, please be sure to take action on what you've learned here, the advice here is simple but golden and has worked for many people, and it can work for you to if you stick to it.

Good luck!

Bonus Report: How To Pick the Perfect Shoe

Welcome To How To Pick The Perfect Shoe

Most people are unaware that there are 3 common foot types and in 3 shoe types to match, and if your shoes don't match your foot type than your feet don't get the support they need and injuries are practically bound to happen.

In this special report you're going to learn the secrets to choosing the perfect shoe to match your feet and give them the support they need.

Why Choosing The Right Shoe Is Vital

It's important that you understand why choosing the right shoe is so important. But instead of telling you about all the delicate tendons, ligaments and muscles that could potentially get stretched, strained, torn or otherwise injured as a result of not having the right type of support, I'll tell you about just a handful of the nasty injuries that arise from such shenanigans.

1. Shin Splints
2. Plantar Fascitis
3. Achilles Tendon Inflammation
4. Posterior Tibialis Syndrome
5. Knee Pains
6. Stress Fractures
7. Heel Spurs

If you don't know what half of those things are, that's great, let's keep it that way!

Read this short report in its entirety and take action on it, and you'll be able to avoid all those nasty injuries and kickass and take names in your chosen sport or activity.

Let's get into it…

How To Identify Your Foot Type

Before you are off to your favourite running store, test yourself and establish your foot type by doing the simple "wet foot" test. Also, refer to the diagram below.

- Wet your foot in the shower, step onto a piece of clean paper.

 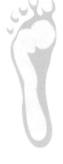

SUPINATOR
Foot doesn't roll over before toe-off, but rolls to the side

NEUTRAL
Ideal biodynamics — no overpronation

OVERPRONATOR
Foot rolls in excessively during the foot strike

- Outline the mark that your foot makes on the paper.

- Finally, make sure to take it with you to the shoe store as it will help in selecting the right shoe.

Type 1: Normal arch (the middle picture)

Your one of the lucky ones; you are a normal pronator and you won't have many problems with your feet. Running shoe shopping for your feet should not be hard. Ask for a **good stability shoe** which offers moderate pronation. Stability shoes offer a good blend of cushioning and support. Lighter runners may prefer neutral-cushioned shoes without any added support, or even a performance training shoe that offers some support but a low profile, for a faster feel.

Type 2: Flat foot (the right picture)

When a flat foot shows, you are overpronating. Your arch collapses inward. Your foot moves too much and this can cause injuries. Therefore you are best of with **motion-control shoes** and good quality insoles. Motion control shoes will prevent your foot from rolling in too far, have a straight shape that gives maximum support to your foot and are the most rigid, control-oriented running shoes.

Type 3: High arch (the left picture)

When there is almost no arch to be seen you are under pronating. Your arch does not collapse enough, thereby causing the shock of your foot landing on the ground to travel upwards to your legs. This can cause injuries.

You should look for a **cushioned shoe**. Cushioned shoes have a curved shape and a softer midsole with the least medial support, which encourages motion and allows your feet to roll inward, hence absorbing shock.

Types Of Shoes

So, depending on your foot type you will need shoes which offer stability, motion control or cushioning:

Motion Control Shoe: Runners with flat feet normally overpronate, so they do well in a **motion-control** shoe that controls pronation.

Stability Shoe: If you have a normal arch, you're likely a **normal pronator**, meaning you'll do best in a normal shoe. A little extra stability is always good, so look for a **stability shoe** that offers moderate pronation control.

There is a common misconception that shoes that are stable are not cushioned. While it is true that stable shoes may be firmer in certain areas of the midsole (this is what helps provide the stability), supportive shoes have just as much cushioning as a shoe labeled "Cushion".

Cushioned Shoe: High-arched runners typically underpronate, so they do best in a **cushioned shoe**

that encourages a more natural foot motion. They should avoid motion control and stability shoes because they prevent the motion that were trying to encourage.

Still Uncertain About Which Shoe To Choose?

If you don't know your foot type or if you are uncertain about it, always visit a specialty running store where they have a **podobaroscope**, a glass surface with a mirror underneath, or where they do **footscan** which will be able to tell you right away what type of foot you have and what type of running shoe you need.

How To Choose The Right Specialty Shoe Store

For the purchase of your shoes always visit a specialty store where they have the proper equipment and expert personnel to help you. It's worth putting in the effort to find a specialist shoe store that you always go to and a store assistant who knows his stuff that you can trust.

Tips For Picking Out A Good Shoe Store:

- They will ask to look at your running shoes, particularly the wear and tear patterns. An expert

- will be able to tell quite a lot about your feet from this.
- They will ask lots of questions about your training and exercise history.
- There is often foot scan equipment or a treadmill with video equipment. This helps the salesman determine which shoes will suit your feet and running style best.
- You are allowed to do a test run; if not on the treadmill, then at least in front of the store. You can't test your shoes properly if you are not allowed to run on them before buying them.
- The staff will be able to tell you how long the shoes will last for. Good running shoes go normally for about 1000km. But there are exceptions, a good shoe store assistant knows which shoes go longer and which don't.

Note: the store I recommend most if you can find one in your area is called "Fleet Feet", they've got expert staff and excellent equipment.

My Shoe Recommendations:

Mizuno Wave Legend
Adidas Calibrate
Brooks Beast
New Balance 1122
New Balance 1220

Nike Air Structure Triax
Saucony Grid Stabhli
Asics Gel MC
Asics Gel Kayano
Asics Gel Koji GS

You've probably noticed I haven't recommend shoes for each foot type, the simple reason why is that I believe it's best for you to go to a running store and get an expert to help you in person, but if you're in need of a good cushion shoe, you'd be hard pressed to find one better then the Brooks Beast... that's the one I use!

Made in United States
Troutdale, OR
10/27/2023

14054995R10033